T0320719

Cambridge Elements ≡

Elements in Emergency Neurosurgery
edited by
Nihal Gurusinghe
Lancashire Teaching Hospital NHS Trust
Peter Hutchinson
University of Cambridge, Society of British Neurological Surgeons and Royal College of Surgeons of England
Ioannis Fouyas
Royal College of Surgeons of Edinburgh
Naomi Slator
North Bristol NHS Trust
Ian Kamaly-Asl
Royal Manchester Children's Hospital
Peter Whitfield
University Hospitals Plymouth NHS Trust

MANAGEMENT OF SEIZURES IN NEUROSURGICAL PRACTICE

Julie Woodfield
Birmingham Children's Hospital
Susan Duncan
NHS Lothian

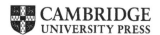

CAMBRIDGE
UNIVERSITY PRESS

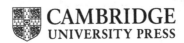

Shaftesbury Road, Cambridge CB2 8EA, United Kingdom

One Liberty Plaza, 20th Floor, New York, NY 10006, USA

477 Williamstown Road, Port Melbourne, VIC 3207, Australia

314–321, 3rd Floor, Plot 3, Splendor Forum, Jasola District Centre, New Delhi – 110025, India

103 Penang Road, #05–06/07, Visioncrest Commercial, Singapore 238467

Cambridge University Press is part of Cambridge University Press & Assessment, a department of the University of Cambridge.

We share the University's mission to contribute to society through the pursuit of education, learning and research at the highest international levels of excellence.

www.cambridge.org
Information on this title: www.cambridge.org/9781009487252

DOI: 10.1017/9781009487238

First published 2024

A catalogue record for this publication is available from the British Library.

ISBN 978-1-009-48725-2 Hardback
ISBN 978-1-009-48724-5 Paperback
ISSN 2755-0656 (online)
ISSN 2755-0648 (print)

Management of Seizures in Neurosurgical Practice

Elements in Emergency Neurosurgery

DOI: 10.1017/9781009487238
First published online: April 2024

Julie Woodfield
Birmingham Children's Hospital

Susan Duncan
NHS Lothian

Author for correspondence: Julie Woodfield, Julie.woodfield@ed.ac.uk

Abstract: Seizures are a presenting feature of many neurosurgical disorders and can arise as a result of neurosurgical treatment or its complications. Recognition and effective management of seizures can be life-saving and will minimise long-term seizure-induced morbidity. In this Element, the authors describe seizure diagnosis, emergency and ongoing management, and considerations in neurosurgical conditions.

Keywords: seizures, epilepsy, anti-epileptic drugs, status epilepticus

ISBNs: 9781009487252 (HB), 9781009487245 (PB), 9781009487238 (OC)
ISSNs: 2755-0656 (online), 2755-0648 (print)

Contents

Introduction

Seizures are a presenting feature of many neurosurgical disorders and can arise as a result of neurosurgical treatment or its complications. Recognition and effective management of seizures can be life-saving and will minimise long-term seizure-induced morbidity. In this Element we describe seizure diagnosis, emergency and ongoing management, and considerations in neurosurgical conditions.

What Is a Seizure?

A seizure is defined as "a transient occurrence of signs and/or symptoms due to abnormal excessive or synchronous neuronal activity in the brain" (1). These bursts of synchronous electrical activity affect brain function. Seizures may present with alterations in sensory, motor, or autonomic function. There may also be altered awareness, cognition, memory, and behaviour (1). Seizures are temporary, with a defined start and end point (1).

Seizures can result from neurosurgical disorders, their complications, or their management. Seizures may be associated with hyponatraemia, hypoglycaemia, intracranial haemorrhage, central nervous system infection, pneumocephalus, or hydrocephalus. It can sometimes be unclear whether an event is a seizure. Clinical events that may mimic seizures or be confused with seizures include: hydrocephalic attacks, new focal neurological deficits, syncope, ischaemic events, dystonia, drug reactions or withdrawal, panic attacks, or features of pre-existing neurological disorders such as migraine aura. Pointers that an event is a seizure include:

- A discrete event with a start and end point
- Progress of symptoms and signs within seconds after onset
- Tongue biting or urinary incontinence
- Desaturation or cyanosis
- Déjà vu sensation or other aura prior to onset
- Occurrence during sleep
- Post-ictal confusion and tiredness lasting hours
- Significant injury during the event such as a vertebral fracture or shoulder dislocation

When it is not clear if events are seizures, videoing the events on a mobile phone and recording an electroencephalogram (EEG) during the events can be helpful. A neurologist should be consulted if there is doubt about whether the events are seizures.

Seizure Types

Classification and description of seizures facilitates communication between healthcare professionals, patients, their families, and carers. Seizure classification plays an important role in guiding investigations and management decisions, understanding prognosis and response to anti-seizure medication, and in teaching and research. The 2017 International League Against Epilepsy operational classification of seizures is shown in Figure 1 (2).

Seizures are described by their onset, which may be focal, generalised, or unknown. Focal onset seizures originate within one hemisphere, and may have motor, sensory, or other features (2). Generalised onset seizures imply the rapid engagement of bilateral brain networks with bilateral features (2). With focal seizures, there may or may not be impaired awareness, but generalised seizures imply a loss of awareness (2).

The ILAE definition of epilepsy is shown in Box 1. Neurosurgical patients with a structural cause for epilepsy have a high risk of further seizures following an initial seizure. Those with tumours, intracranial haemorrhage, or brain abscesses usually meet this definition of epilepsy and are treated with anti-epileptic drugs (AEDs) following their first seizure.

ILAE 2017 Classification of Seizure Types Expanded Version [1]

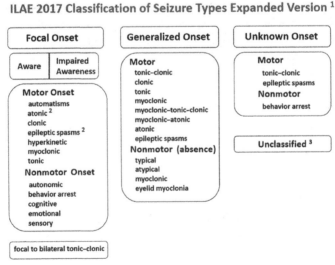

Figure 1 ILAE 2017 classification of seizure types expanded version

1. Definitions, other seizure types, and descriptors are listed in the accompanying paper and glossary of terms.
2. Degree of awareness usually is not specified.
3. Due to inadequate information or inability to place in other categories.

> **Box 1 ILAE 2014 DEFINITION OF EPILEPSY**
>
> Practical clinical definition of epilepsy from the 2014 ILAE position paper (3). Epilepsy is a disease of the brain defined by any of the following conditions:
>
> 1. At least two unprovoked (or reflex) seizures occurring >24 h apart
> 2. One unprovoked (or reflex) seizure and a probability of further seizures similar to the general recurrence risk (at least 60%) after two unprovoked seizures, occurring over the next 10 years
> 3. Diagnosis of an epilepsy syndrome

Epilepsy is considered to be resolved for individuals who had an age-dependent epilepsy syndrome but are now past the applicable age or those who have remained seizure free for the last 10 years, with no seizure medicines for the last 5 years.

Management of Seizures

Emergency Seizure Management

All episodes of unresponsiveness should be managed using an ABC approach to resuscitation. Emergency resuscitation and treatment should be started whilst assessing for reversible causes and prior to establishing a definitive diagnosis of seizure activity. Figure 2 shows an algorithm for the emergency management of seizures. Ambulant patients may be outside their bedspace at the time of a seizure, and their environment should be made safe to prevent injury and facilitate ongoing management.

Manual airway manoeuvres and airway adjuncts may be required. If a seizing patient is jaw clenching, a nasopharyngeal airway is easier to insert and will maintain the airway. However, a nasopharyngeal airway may be contraindicated following trauma to the nasal sinuses and skull base. Always give oxygen; seizures are associated with desaturation. The recovery position may be the safest position, but in patients with spinal trauma, this may not be possible as spinal alignment may need to be preserved and turning may require log rolling. Intravenous access should be established, and bloods sent. A full blood count, urea and electrolytes, coagulation screen, and blood transfusion sample should be sent to investigate the cause of the seizure, and in preparation for any required surgical intervention. The quickest haemoglobin and sodium levels will be available on a venous blood gas. The bedside glucose should be checked

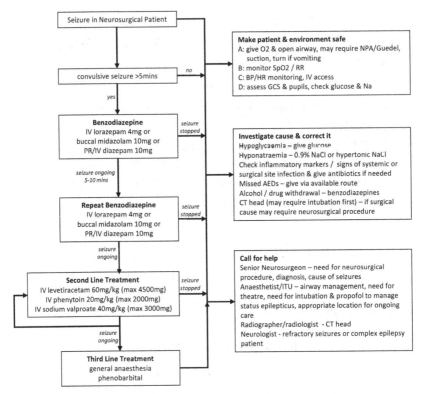

Figure 2 Seizure management in neurosurgical patients

The three boxes for making the patient safe, investigating the cause, and calling for help should be considered simultaneously. They are applicable at all stages of the treatment pathway. Doses given are for adults. Refer to the BNF and local guidelines for safety and administration considerations. (NPA, nasopharyngeal airway; RR, respiratory rate, BP, blood pressure; HR, heart rate; GCS, Glasgow Coma Scale; Na, sodium; NaCl, sodium chloride; AED, anti-epileptic drug; CT, computed tomography; IV, intravenous; PR, per rectum)

to ensure the patient is not hypoglycaemic. Hypoglycaemia is particularly a risk in those unable to eat, for example, due to being nil by mouth pre-operatively, those with post-operative nausea and vomiting, or those with a low conscious level, or brainstem or lower cranial nerve pathologies affecting swallowing. Imaging with a CT head to assess for surgically reversible causes should be considered in every neurosurgical patient with new onset seizures. This may require anaesthetic support or intubation and ventilation prior to transfer to the CT scanner.

Causes of seizures to consider in neurosurgical patients include:
- Hypoglycaemia
- Hyponatraemia
- Hypoxia
- Raised intracranial pressure
- Hydrocephalus or blocked ventriculoperitoneal shunt
- Central nervous system infection
- Cerebral oedema
- Space occupying lesion
- Intracranial haemorrhage
- Stroke or cerebral ischaemia
- Drug or toxin ingestion or withdrawal
- Missed or incorrectly prescribed or administered AEDs

Hyponatraemia is common following traumatic brain injury (TBI) and subarachnoid haemorrhage (SAH) and should be treated with slow correction of the serum sodium to avoid further seizures. Causes of seizures such as acute hydrocephalus, or post-operative haematoma or infection will require surgical treatment.

Status Epilepticus

Status epilepticus is defined as prolonged seizures lasting more than thirty minutes or recurrent seizures without a return to baseline between seizures (4). Guidelines advise treatment for anyone with convulsive seizures lasting five minutes or more (4). Intravenous lorazepam is first line in the hospital setting when intravenous access is available, but buccal midazolam or rectal diazepam may be given when intravenous access is not immediately possible. If the seizure does not stop within five to ten minutes, a further dose of benzodiazepine should be administered. If convulsive status epilepticus does not respond to two doses of a benzodiazepine, then second-line treatment with levetiracetam, phenytoin, or sodium valproate should be given. If this is not successful, one of the alternative second-line treatments can be tried. Third-line options are general anaesthesia and phenobarbital, so discussion with the senior neurosurgeon, a neurologist, an anaesthetist, and the intensive care unit should occur (4).

The Advanced Paediatric Life Support algorithm for management of paediatric seizures is shown in Figure 3. Those who are under consideration for epilepsy surgery or who have known refractory epilepsy may have individualised emergency management plans to follow in the event of refractory seizures. Guidance from a neurologist is also very helpful for those suspected to be in non-convulsive status epilepticus and those with ongoing focal seizures, clusters of seizures, or complex medication-resistant epilepsy.

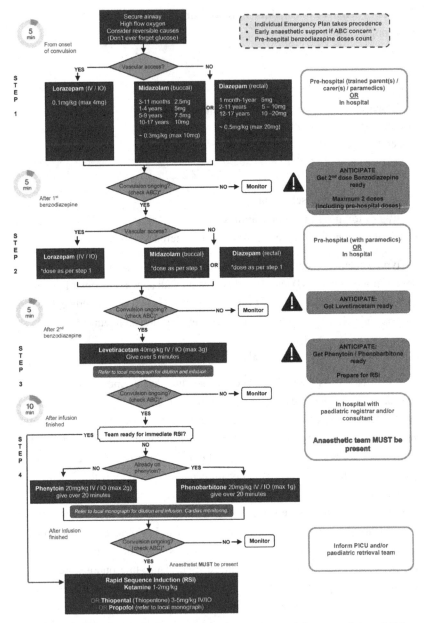

Figure 3 APLS 2021 Algorithm for management of the convulsing child

Anti-epileptic Drugs

Recommended treatment options for generalised tonic clonic seizures are levetiracetam or lamotrigine in women who can bear children and sodium valproate in men, girls under the age of ten, girls who are unlikely to need sodium valproate after they reach childbearing age, and women who cannot bear children (4). For focal seizures, lamotrigine or levetiracetam is the first-line monotherapy, with carbamazepine, oxcarbazepine, and zonisamide as second-line treatments (4). Levetiracetam and phenytoin are often used for seizures with a neurosurgical cause. Commonly used anti-epileptics and considerations for prescribing in neurosurgical patients are shown in Table 1. Sodium valproate is not given to women of childbearing age because up to four in ten babies are at risk of developmental disorders and approximately one in ten are at risk of birth defects if valproate is used in pregnancy (5).

Seizures and Neurosurgical Conditions
Traumatic Brain Injury and Seizures

Seizures occur in up to 15 per cent of people following a TBI, and may be associated with a poorer prognosis or complications (6). Seizures following TBI are classified as immediate (within twenty-four hours of injury), early (within one week of injury), and late (more than one week following injury) (6, 7). Meta-analyses suggest anticonvulsants reduce the rate of early, but not late, post-traumatic seizures (6, 7). Brain Trauma Foundation Guidelines recommend prophylactic AED treatment to decrease the incidence of early post-traumatic seizures when the overall benefit is felt to outweigh the complications associated with treatment (8). Although levetiracetam may be theoretically favoured over phenytoin due to its better side effect profile and lack of need for blood monitoring, systematic reviews do not show an advantage in side effect frequency (9), and Brain Trauma Foundation Guidelines state that there is insufficient evidence to recommend levetiracetam over phenytoin (8). When AEDs are given for post-traumatic seizure prophylaxis, a one- or two-week course at full dose is usually given without weaning the dose up or down.

Tumour Surgery and Seizures

Up to 60 per cent of those with a brain tumour will have a seizure at some time (10). Low-grade lesions tend to be more epileptogenic, and complete resection of a low-grade lesion can give seizure freedom rates up to 85 per cent in epilepsy surgery programmes (10). There is no compelling evidence that treatment with AEDs prevents the development of seizures, and guidelines recommend that in the absence of seizures, there is no role for prophylactic AEDs, even for those undergoing neurosurgical procedures (11, 12). There is no robust evidence that the use of levetiracetam or sodium valproate prolongs survival in those with gliomas (11, 12). However, seizure control can affect quality of life, and in those

Table 1 AEDs in neurosurgical practice

AED	Usage notes	Side effects
Lorazepam	First-line IV to terminate seizure	Respiratory depression, drowsiness, agitation
Diazepam (Diazemuls-emulsion for injection)	PR or IV to terminate seizure Oral tablets used to manage alcohol withdrawal, anxiety, etc. (e.g. facilitate MRI scanning)	Respiratory depression, drowsiness, agitation
Midazolam (Buccolam/Epistatus)	Buccal oral gel to terminate seizure	Respiratory depression, drowsiness, agitation, vomiting
Levetiracetam (Keppra)	Loading dose (60 mg/kg IV, up to 4.5 g) for status epilepticus, then maintenance dose	Anxiety, mood/behaviour alteration – "Keppra rage," decreased appetite, skin reactions, vertigo, vomiting
Phenytoin (Dilantin/Epanutin)	Loading dose (20 mg/kg, up to 2 g) for status epilepticus, then maintenance dose Oral and IV doses may not be equivalent Requires IV filter on giving set, cardiac monitoring, blood level monitoring, avoid in pregnancy	Cardiovascular instability and arrhythmias (do not give in heart block), rash and skin reactions, extravasation and injection necrosis, respiratory disorders, seizures, abnormal blood counts, gingival hyperplasia, lip swelling, nephritis, paraesthesia, vomiting Phenytoin toxicity: nystagmus, diplopia, slurred speech, ataxia, confusion, hyperglycaemia

Drug	Notes	Side effects
Sodium valproate/ valproic acid (Epilim/Depakote/ Depakin/Dyzantil/ Epival/Episenta)	Long acting forms not equivalent to short acting forms Do not give to women or girls able to have children unless pregnancy prevention programme in place May be discontinued prior to neurosurgical procedures due to risk of bleeding with platelet dysfunction	Platelet dysfunction, thrombocytopaenia, dizziness, alopecia, anaemia, abnormal behaviour/concentration, deafness, hyponatraemia, nail disorders, nausea, abdominal pain, weight gain, teratogenic
Lamotrigine (Lamictal)	Avoid abrupt withdrawal	Suicidal thoughts, aggression, agitation, diarrhoea, rash, nausea and vomiting, sleep disorders, skin reactions
Carbamazepine (Tegretol)	Used for focal seizures Used for trigeminal neuralgia	Hyponatraemia, dizziness, drowsiness, dry mouth, fatigue, vomiting, weight gain, abdominal pain, headache, oedema, skin reactions, blurred vision
Clobazam (Frisium/ Perizam/Tapclob/ Zacco)	Add-on drug, used in medication-resistant epilepsy when neurosurgery may provoke seizures	Drowsiness, aggression, respiratory depression, dysarthria, nystagmus, headache, hypotension, muscle weakness, nausea, tremor, withdrawal

Generic names are given with brand or other names are in brackets. Only common or neurosurgically relevant side effects are shown. For a full list of side effects and dosing information, consult the British National Formulary. (AED, anti-epileptic drug; IV, intravenous)

with seizures and a brain tumour, AEDs should be started, and are usually prescribed following a single seizure (12).

Intracranial Infection and Seizures

One-third of those with a brain abscess will develop epilepsy (13). Although some authors recommend three to six months of treatment with AEDs for those with brain abscesses, there is little evidence to support this strategy (13). Post-operative cranial infectious complications may also cause seizures, and both AEDs and antimicrobials should be given in this scenario (14).

Vascular Disorders and Seizures

In SAH, seizures may occur at onset or be associated with complications such as hyponatraemia, hydrocephalus, re-bleeding, or delayed ischaemic neurological deficit (15). There are no randomised controlled trials of primary or secondary prevention of seizures following SAH (16), and the use of seizure prophylaxis varies worldwide (15). When seizures occur after the time of ictus, they are usually treated with AEDs, but any associated complications such as hydrocephalus or hyponatraemia should also be managed to prevent further seizures.

Following intracranial haemorrhage, seizures occur in up to 30 per cent (17), and 90 per cent of those who have had one seizure will have a further seizure (18). Haemorrhagic stroke guidelines do not recommend prophylactic treatment with AEDs, but AEDs should be started if seizures occur, although they do not reduce the risk of late seizures (19, 20).

Epilepsy Surgery

Patients with medication-resistant epilepsy may be admitted to neurosurgery and neurology wards for investigation and surgical management of their epilepsy. Video EEG using scalp electrodes or implantable depth or subdural electrodes, ictal SPECT, vagal nerve stimulator insertion or battery changes, or disconnective or resective surgical procedures may all be carried out. Patients are usually taking at least two AEDs and may take significantly more. It is important to ensure that patients with epilepsy have their AEDs prescribed and given at the correct times via the correct routes, or alternative dose and route adjustments are made peri-operatively. Those with medication-resistant epilepsy may have personalised seizure plans and these should be easily available, consulted, and followed if seizures occur. Personal plans may differ significantly from standard treatment. For investigative procedures, AED withdrawal may be planned. There should always be a plan available regarding medications for seizures during drug withdrawal. Discussion with the named neurologist and neurosurgeon is crucial for these patients to ensure that the most information is gleaned regarding epilepsy onset in the safest possible way. Do not hesitate to seek senior support from neurologists and neurosurgeons for patients with known medication-resistant epilepsy who are having seizures.

Patients who are under investigation for non-epileptic attacks may also be admitted for video telemetry. Again, a personalised treatment and seizure plan should be in place. There may be a decision in place not to treat seizures in some instances whilst investigation is ongoing, but this should be confirmed with the treating neurology team. You should always provide emergency resuscitation and life-saving treatment by managing the airway, breathing, and circulation and ensuring the patient is safe.

Considerations for Discharge

Except for short-term prophylactic treatment, AEDs should not be stopped abruptly. Patients started on AEDs should be advised to continue them until outpatient review with neurology or neurosurgery, when a personalised weaning plan can be created if it is appropriate to wean the AEDs.

Epilepsy is associated with an increased risk of premature death, including sudden unexpected death in epilepsy (SUDEP). Patients and their families should be advised that SUDEP is associated with non-adherence to medication, alcohol and drug misuse, living alone, sleeping alone without supervision, having uncontrolled seizures, and having generalised tonic-clonic seizures, and the risks are higher in those with a previous brain injury, previous central nervous system infection, metastatic cancer, previous stroke, and abnormal neurological examination findings (21). Support and arrangements for managing these risks should be discussed. Referral to an epilepsy specialist nurse with experience in discussing and managing risks around the house, at work, and when out and about is helpful for patients with a new diagnosis of epilepsy. Updating the usual epilepsy team for any patients with long-standing epilepsy admitted for a neurosurgical procedure is essential for continuity of care.

People with epilepsy must inform the Driver and Vehicle Licensing Agency in the UK. Rules surrounding driving licences will depend on the seizure type and frequency, any neurosurgical procedure performed, and the underlying condition.

Neurosurgical Cases

Scenario 1

You are the junior doctor covering the neurosurgical ward in the evening. You are called urgently to review a fifty-four-year-old woman who has been having a generalised tonic-clonic seizure for over five minutes. The nursing staff have placed a nasopharyngeal airway and are administering high flow oxygen. The patient has been placed in the recovery position. She had been receiving fluids through a cannula at the time of the seizure, and the cannula is still in place and has been flushed and is working. The nursing staff tell you the patient was admitted that morning following a sudden onset headache. A CT scan showed an SAH, and the patient was transferred to the neurosurgical ward. Her Glasgow Coma Scale (GCS) score was 15 with no focal neurological deficit prior to the seizure but had been vomiting and had a severe headache.

- How do you manage this scenario?

  Assess the patient using an ABC approach.

  ○ A: Check the airway is patent and maintained with the nasopharyngeal airway
  ○ B: Check the patient is breathing, and check SpO_2 and respiratory rate
  ○ C: Check the pulse, blood pressure, and capillary refill
  ○ D: Check glucose, GCS, and pupils, and assess for ongoing seizure activity

Manage any ABC concerns, and administer IV lorazepam if the seizure is still ongoing.

- What is the likely cause for the seizure?

  The possible causes are:

  ○ Aneurysm re-bleed
  ○ Hydrocephalus
  ○ Hyponatraemia (due to vomiting or SAH)
  ○ Hypoglycaemia (due to vomiting and poor oral intake)

Hypoglycaemia can be assessed using a bedside test or a blood gas. Serum sodium can be assessed using a blood gas. A CT head is required to diagnose a re-bleed or hydrocephalus. Therefore, you need to take a blood gas, bloods, and arrange a CT head.

Following the IV lorazepam, the patient has stopped seizing but is now drowsy, with a GCS of E1V1M4. Her respiratory rate is low. To safely arrange a CT head, you call the anaesthetist, the neurosurgery registrar, and the radiologist. The anaesthetist intubates and ventilates the patient and transfers them safely to CT. The CT head shows hydrocephalus (Figure 4).

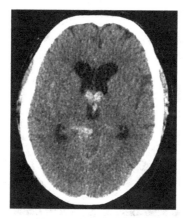

Figure 4 CT head – scenario 1

CT head showing hydrocephalus due to subarachnoid and intraventricular haemorrhage.

The neurosurgeon takes the patient to theatre for insertion of an external ventricular drain. The patient is woken up at the end of the procedure and returns to a GCS of E4V4M6. She is not started on any anti-epileptic medications and has no further seizures during her hospital stay.

Scenario 2

You are the junior doctor on the neurosurgery ward, and you are called to see a thirty-five-year-old man regarding his arm symptoms. The nurses think he is having a focal seizure. He has been an inpatient for a week following aspiration of a left frontal abscess secondary to sinusitis. He is on appropriate intravenous antibiotics. You assess him and find he has uncontrollable rhythmic jerking movements of his right arm. He is speaking to you and can tell you that it started half an hour ago and he has been unable to control his arm since. He has no other symptoms. What do you do?

You call the neurosurgery registrar for advice, who suggests giving a loading dose of levetiracetam and organising a CT scan. The seizure settles within ten minutes of giving levetiracetam. You reassess the patient, who is GCS 15 with normal observations and is no longer having a seizure. You decide it is safe for you to accompany him to CT. The CT shows an increase in the size of the abscess (Figure 5).

The patient returns to theatre for re-aspiration of the abscess. Because there is a high risk of further seizures, you prescribe him regular levetiracetam after discussing with the neurosurgeon. This patient has further focal seizures over the next weeks, but these are successfully treated with an increasing dose of

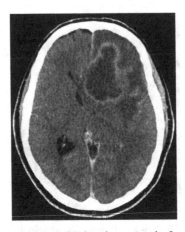

Figure 5 CT head – scenario 2

CT head showing left frontal abscess with midline shift.

levetiracetam. He is kept on levetiracetam for the duration of his antibiotic treatment (three months). After this time, a discussion about the risks and benefits of continuing versus stopping the levetiracetam can be held between the patient and an epilepsy specialist (see the "Intracranial Infection and Seizures" section).

References

1. Fisher RS, van Emde Boas W, Blume W, et al. Epileptic Seizures and Epilepsy: Definitions Proposed by the International League Against Epilepsy (ILAE) and the International Bureau for Epilepsy (IBE). *Epilepsia.* 2005;46(4):470–2.

2. Fisher RS, Cross JH, French JA, et al. Operational Classification of Seizure Types by the International League Against Epilepsy: Position Paper of the ILAE Commission for Classification and Terminology. *Epilepsia.* 2017;58 (4):522–30.

3. Fisher RS, Acevedo C, Arzimanoglou A, et al. ILAE Official Report: A Practical Clinical Definition of Epilepsy. *Epilepsia.* 2014;55(4):475–82.

4. NICE NIfHaCE. Epilepsies in Children, Young people and Adults. 27 April 2022.

5. Medicines and Healthcare Products Regulatory Agency. Valproate Use by Women and Girls. UK Government Report. 2018.

6. Wilson CD, Burks JD, Rodgers RB, et al. Early and Late Posttraumatic Epilepsy in the Setting of Traumatic Brain Injury: A Meta-analysis and Review of Antiepileptic Management. *World Neurosurgery.* 2018;110:e901–6.

7. Thompson K, Pohlmann-Eden B, Campbell LA, Abel H. Pharmacological Treatments for Preventing Epilepsy Following Traumatic Head Injury. *Cochrane Database of Systematic Reviews.* 2015(8). doi: 10.1002/14651858 .CD009900.pub2.

8. Carney N, Totten AM, O'Reilly C, et al. Guidelines for the Management of Severe Traumatic Brain Injury. 2016. Contract No.: 4th ed. Neurosurgery 2017 Jan 1;80(1):6–15. doi: 10.1227/NEU.0000000000001432.

9. Zhao L, Wu YP, Qi JL, et al. Efficacy of Levetiracetam Compared with Phenytoin in Prevention of Seizures in Brain Injured Patients: A Meta-analysis. *Medicine* (Baltimore). 2018;97(48):e13247.

10. Chen DY, Chen CC, Crawford JR, Wang SG. Tumor-related Epilepsy: Epidemiology, Pathogenesis and Management. *Journal of Neuro-Oncology.* 2018;139(1):13–21.

11. Walbert T, Harrison RA, Schiff D, et al. SNO and EANO Practice Guideline Update: Anticonvulsant Prophylaxis in Patients with Newly Diagnosed Brain Tumors. *Neuro-Oncology.* 2021;23(11):1835–44.

12. Weller M, van den Bent M, Preusser M, et al. EANO Guidelines on the Diagnosis and Treatment of Diffuse Gliomas of Adulthood. *Nature Reviews Clinical Oncology.* 2021;18(3):170–86.

13. Bodilsen J, Dalager-Pedersen M, van de Beek D, Brouwer MC, Nielsen H. Long-term Mortality and Epilepsy in Patients After Brain Abscess: A Nationwide Population-Based Matched Cohort Study. *Clinical Infectious Diseases.* 2020;71(11):2825–32.
14. Ersoy TF, Ridwan S, Grote A, Coras R, Simon M. Early Postoperative Seizures (EPS) in Patients Undergoing Brain Tumour Surgery. *Scientific Reports.* 2020;10(1):13674.
15. Lanzino G, D'Urso PI, Suarez J. Seizures and Anticonvulsants After Aneurysmal Subarachnoid Hemorrhage. *Neurocritical Care.* 2011;15(2): 247–56.
16. Marigold R, Günther A, Tiwari D, Kwan J. Antiepileptic Drugs for the Primary and Secondary Prevention of Seizures After Subarachnoid Haemorrhage. *Cochrane Database of Systematic Reviews.* 2013;2013(6): Cd008710.
17. Steiner T, Kaste M, Forsting M, et al. Recommendations for the Management of Intracranial Haemorrhage – Part I: Spontaneous Intracerebral Haemorrhage. The European Stroke Initiative Writing Committee and the Writing Committee for the EUSI Executive Committee. *Cerebrovascular Diseases.* 2006;22(4):294–316.
18. Haapaniemi E, Strbian D, Rossi C, et al. The CAVE Score for Predicting Late Seizures After Intracerebral Hemorrhage. *Stroke.* 2014;45(7):1971–6.
19. Greenberg SM, Ziai WC, Cordonnier C, et al. Guideline for the Management of Patients with Spontaneous Intracerebral Hemorrhage: A Guideline from the American Heart Association/American Stroke Association. *Stroke.* 2022;53(7):e282–e361.
20. Steiner T, Al-Shahi Salman R, Beer R, et al. European Stroke Organisation (ESO) Guidelines for the Management of Spontaneous Intracerebral Hemorrhage. *International Journal of Stroke.* 2014;9(7):840–55.
21. National Institute for Health and Care Excellence. Epilepsies in Children, Young People, and Adults. 2022. https://www.nice.org.uk/guidance/ng217 27 April 2022.

Cambridge Elements ⹀

Emergency Neurosurgery

Nihal Gurusinghe

Lancashire Teaching Hospital NHS Trust

Professor Nihal Gurusinghe is a Consultant Neurosurgeon at the Lancashire Teaching Hospitals NHS Trust. He is on the Executive Council of the Society of British Neurological Surgeons as the Lead for NICE (National Institute for Health and Care Excellence) guidelines relating to neurosurgical practice. He is also an examiner for the UK and International FRCS examinations in Neurosurgery.

Peter Hutchinson

University of Cambridge, Society of British Neurological Surgeons and Royal College of Surgeons of England

Peter Hutchinson BSc MBBS FFSEM FRCS(SN) PhD FMedSci is Professor of Neurosurgery and Head of the Division of Academic Neurosurgery at the University of Cambridge, and Honorary Consultant Neurosurgeon at Addenbrooke's Hospital. He is Director of Clinical Research at the Royal College of Surgeons of England and Meetings Secretary of the Society of British Neurological Surgeons.

Ioannis Fouyas

Royal College of Surgeons of Edinburgh

Ioannis Fouyas is a Consultant Neurosurgeon in Edinburgh. His clinical interests focus on the treatment of complex cerebrovascular and skull base pathologies. His academic endeavours concentrate in the field of cerebrovascular pathophysiology. His passion is technical surgical training, fulfilled in collaboration with the Royal College of Surgeons of Edinburgh. Finally, he pursues Undergraduate Neuroscience teaching, with a particular focus on functional Neuroanatomy.

Naomi Slator

North Bristol NHS Trust

Naomi Slator FRCS (SN) is a Consultant Spinal Neurosurgeon based at North Bristol NHS Trust. She has a specialist interest in Complex Spine alongside Cranial and Spinal Trauma. She completed her neurosurgical training in Birmingham and a six-month Fellowship in CSF and Trauma (2019). She then went on to complete her Spinal Fellowship in Leeds (2020) before moving to the southwest to take up her consultant post.

Ian Kamaly-Asl

Royal Manchester Children's Hospital

Ian Kamaly-Asl is a full time paediatric neurosurgeon and Honorary Chair at Royal Manchester Children's Hospital. He trained in North Western Deanery with fellowships at Boston Children's Hospital and Sick Kids in Toronto. Ian is a member of council of The Royal College of Surgeons of England and The SBNS where he is lead for mentoring and tackling oppressive behaviours.

Peter Whitfield

University Hospitals Plymouth NHS Trust

Professor Peter Whitfield is a Consultant Neurosurgeon at the South West Neurosurgical Centre, University Hospitals Plymouth NHS Trust. His clinical interests include vascular neurosurgery, neuro oncology and trauma. He has held many roles in postgraduate neurosurgical education and is President of the Society of British Neurological Surgeons. Peter has published widely, and is passionate about education, training and the promotion of clinical research.

About the Series

Elements in Emergency Neurosurgery is intended for trainees and practitioners in Neurosurgery and Emergency Medicine as well as allied specialties all over the world. Authored by international experts, this series provides core knowledge, common clinical pathways and recommendations on the management of acute conditions of the brain and spine.

Cambridge Elements ☰

Emergency Neurosurgery

Elements in the Series

Printed in the United States
by Baker & Taylor Publisher Services